Mediterranean Diet for Beginners:

All you Need to Know About Mediterranean Diet in Simple Guide to Help you Lose Weight Easily. + Simple Recipes for Every Day! Weight Loss Solution!

render any resulting actions solely under their purview. There are no scenarios in which the publisher or the original author of this work can be in any fashion deemed liable for any hardship or damages that may befall them after undertaking information described herein.

Additionally, the information in the following pages is intended only for informational purposes and should thus be thought of as universal. As befitting its nature, it is presented without assurance regarding its prolonged validity or interim quality. Trademarks that are mentioned are done without written consent and can in no way be considered an endorsement from the trademark holder.

Disclaimer

All content in this book including images, text, and all other formats are provided for informational purposes only. It is not intended, in any way, to be a substitute for the professional medical diagnosis, treatment, or advice. You should always seek medical advice from a healthcare professional with any question you may have regarding a medical condition.

Table of Contents

Chapter one: Introduction

There are many diets that are gaining traction over the past few years as everyone is wanting to be the best versions of themselves that they can possibly be. One diet in particular that has gained a lot of this attention is the Mediterranean diet. Unlike other diets that boast healthy benefits but have very bad side effects, the Mediterranean diet boasts that it can bring you healthy benefits without as many side effects. An important thing to remember however is this book is just a guide to the Mediterranean diet and we are in no way a substitute for a doctor, nutritionist or an official person that has a degree in such matters. As with anything else you should check with your doctor or nutritionist first to make sure that this is a diet that will work for your body and your specific needs. Another reason you should check with your doctor or your nutritionist is everybody has different health issues and so everyone would experience different results as no two people are alike.

Unlike other diet's that take away food from you and say that you can't eat them, like bread, for example, this diet doesn't have that issue and it actually lets you eat some of those foods that you would be missing in other diets.

The Mediterranean diet is a diet that is inspired by Greece, Spain and certain parts of Italy. The diet focuses on the eating habits of these countries during the 1940s and then again in the 1950s. Obviously, the way we eat, and our health has obviously gained more information in the past 50 years which means that your results may differ, but the Mediterranean diet says that despite these things the health benefits of this diet are beneficial to each and every individual person.

For this diet you would need to eat legumes, unrefined cereals or unrefined fruits, a moderate to high consumption of fish, you would also need to eat vegetables and a high consumption of olive oil. You should only have a moderate consumption of all dairy products and a low consumption of non-fish products that contain meat.

Some of the health benefits of the Mediterranean diet boast is that it said to be able to lower the risk of heart disease which in turn can lower the risk of you dying early. As recent as 3 years ago evidence has found that practicing a Mediterranean diet can lead to less overall cancer incidence and it may help against neurodegenerative diseases or even cardiovascular diseases and diabetes. As early as 2 years ago studies have shown that it can also help reduce the risk of non-communicable diseases. In addition, there is also a correlation between a healthy diet and lowering your risk of depression which means the Mediterranean diet may also help lower risk of depression as well because your being healthy.

The Mediterranean diet also includes products containing gluten. What this means is if you have an increase in this diet which you would if you were using this diet every day, you would not be able to follow this diet if you had a gluten related disorder.

Though this diet is laxer than others it does have foods that you need to avoid in order to make this diet work to its best advantage. You will need to avoid sugars, and this includes refined sugars as well as unrefined sugars. You will also need to stay away from red meat. This is a huge thing with a Mediterranean diet as the only need that they really want you to consume is high portions of fish. If you have to consume other meat you should eat it in low portions.

In addition, you should stay away from refined grains like white bread, though other breads are allowed. You should also avoid trans fats and refined oils such as soybean oil or canola oil. For the Mediterranean diet, you mostly want to stick with olive oil.

Another thing that you want to avoid on the Mediterranean diet is processed meats and processed foods. Processed foods are pretty much everywhere you go and any time you look in a supermarket there are rows upon rows of processed foods. This diet is strict in the fact that it wants you to eat more natural foods instead of highly processed foods and in all honesty, most of the other diets that you would find yourself wanting to try are the same way. The Mediterranean diet stresses this because in order to get the best results you need to stay away from food that's going to harm your body. Processed meats such as sausages or hot dogs are another thing that you should avoid on this diet as well. Instead, you should check your labels and make sure that you're eating healthy instead of making choices for your food simply for convenience or cost efficiency. Cost is very important for any diet but remember, it's not more important than your health.

Research, however, shows that some people that are benefiting from the diet have a slightly larger advantage than others who are trying this diet and not succeeding. Research in Italy and in the United States has shown that people who have a higher income may benefit more from this diet than families who don't have as much income to spend. The reason behind this is that people who have a higher income are able to buy a higher quality of product whereas people with lower income don't necessarily have the ability to spend as much money, so they have to buy the lower quality products.

A good example that the study uses is olive oil. Now as we stated before olive oil is an important part of this diet and they want you to consume it as your key oil. An upper-class family would be able to afford a bottle that could cost $10 or more. For many, that's too expensive for a bottle of olive oil because many people don't have a lot of money to spend. There are just as many that think $10 is a cheap price for olive oil. Lower income families, however, would only be able to buy the bottle that's $.97. A bottle that's $.97 might not have the same nutritional value as the bottle that cost $10. There is more research being done on this topic but studies in Italy have been done on over 6,000 people and over a course of a few years they found that more of the lower income families were suffering from heart issues whereas the higher income families were not.

Portion control is also another downside of the Mediterranean diet. As most of the things that you will read online or in a book do not tell you the exact portion size with this book, we tried not to do that as much as other books have. We have also told you the nutritional information as well so that you can get a clear idea of how to do this diet successfully and exactly how much you should be eating. The reason that this is important is that others don't do this, and people tend to consume too much olive oil, or they can assume to many meals and end up over eating. This, in turn, causes harm to the body and the heart.

It is also said that a pregnant woman should be careful on this diet. You should talk to your doctor immediately to make sure that this is alright for you because there are many benefits to being on a Mediterranean diet and studies are trying to discover if those benefits extend to pregnant women and their unborn child as well. Obviously, every pregnant woman is different, and each individual woman has different health needs as well as the unborn child. Therefore, it would be best to talk to your doctor before making any decisions about it when you're pregnant because this book is in no way a substitute for health professional.

Chapter two: Breakfast Recipes

Everyone has heard the expression that breakfast is the most important meal of the day. When you wake up in the morning you need fuel for your day, and you know you're going to need energy because otherwise, you won't be able to function properly during the day. This is where tasty breakfast options come in. When you find yourself missing breakfast you have hunger pains throughout the day. It's your bodies way of telling you, that you need to eat. This diet stresses that you get your main meals in and that you should be consistent.

We have recipes that are quick and easy as well as having multiple servings and it's great because you can reheat these recipes later and it's less cooking if you don't have a lot of time or if you like meal prepping. This saves a lot of time and resources for people, so the recipes are beneficial. The recipes in this chapter are great for breakfast and making sure that you're going to get your fuel for the day and stay energized as well. We want to avoid what is known as the mid-morning slump that people get throughout the day so we will be providing recipes that have what you need to avoid this issue.

These recipes are encouraging healthier eating and the recipes are good nutritionally because of that fact. On the Mediterranean diet, one of the best things is that while you do have to give up some foods because they are unhealthy for you, you can still eat your favorites and enjoy some decadence. For breakfast items, this does mean that were going to have to substitute some items, but the end result is a much healthier diet and a much healthier body.

This recipe is simple and has very few steps making it perfect for people who are beginners at cooking and this diet and people who don't have a lot of time on their hands. Breakfast time is where you need to make sure that your getting your energy to get a good start to your day, but you also need to make sure that having a good breakfast isn't going to cost you getting to work or school on time either.

Frittata

The prep time needed for this recipe is 5 minutes where the cook time will be 20.

This serves 6 people.

Ingredients:

- 1 tsp oregano
- ¼ c of Spanish olives (they will need to be chopped)
- ¼ c of Kalamata olives (they will need to be chopped)
- ½ c tomatoes (they will need to be diced)
- 6 eggs
- ½ c of either cream or milk whichever is the preference for you
- ¼ c of feta (it will need to be crumbled)

Instructions:

- Step one: You need to preheat your oven to 400 degrees exactly.
- Step two: You need a pie pan that is at least 8 inches and then you will need to grease it.
- Step three: Whisk your milk and eggs together until they are blended together.
- Step four: Then you will need to place in your remaining ingredients and mix them together as well.
- Step five: Place in the oven and bake for at least 15 minutes and no later than 20 minutes. Make sure that the eggs are set.

Nutritional information:

This is based on one serving.

Your calories are going to be 107.

Your cholesterol is going to be 169 milligrams.

Your potassium is going to be 130 mg.

Your total fat is going to be 7 grams.

Your sodium is going to be 705 milligrams.

Your protein is going to be 7 grams.

Your total carbohydrates are going to be 3 grams.

Your sugar is going to be 2 grams.

Breakfast bowls are gaining popularity as well and we have a great recipe for one right here. This bowl has quinoa which is a healthy item for any meal. It is also packed full of eggs which means that your protein in this meal is going to be pretty high.

Breakfast Bowl

This recipe takes 10 minutes of prep time while needing 20 minutes

This recipe will serve 6 people

Ingredients:

- 2 c of quinoa (cooked)
- 1 tsp of garlic (granulated)
- 12 eggs
- 1 c of cheese (use feta)
- 1 tsp olive oil
- 1 tsp onion powder
- 1 bag spinach (use baby spinach in a 5 ounce bag)
- ¼ cup yogurt (use Greek and make sure it is plain)
- 1 pint tomatoes (use cherry tomatoes and halve them)

Instructions:

- Step one: Get a bowl and mix your onion powder, garlic, yogurt, and your eggs and then set it aside.
- Step two: Get yourself a skillet and heat your olive oil before adding the spinach.
- Step three: Cook your spinach and make sure that it is wilted a bit. This process should take no more than 4 minutes.
- Step four: Place your tomatoes in as well and cook until they are soft. This should also take no more than 4 minutes.
- Step five: You will now need to stir in the egg mix that you made before and cook until the eggs have set. This should take no longer than 9 minutes. Be sure that while your cooking you stir the eggs so that they will turn out scrambled.
- Step six: When you've made sure that they egg have set, stir in the quinoa and cheese.
- Step seven: Now you need to cook it until its heated through.
- Step eight: You can now serve it and make sure that you serve it hot.

Nutritional Information:

This is based on 1 ¼ of a cup

Your calories are going to be 357.

Your total fat is going to be 20 grams.

Your protein is going to be 23 grams.

Your total carbohydrates are going to be 20 grams.

Your sugar is going to be 4 grams.

Your fiber is going to be 3 grams.

Omelets are a good source of protein for breakfast as well and this omelet has great Mediterranean flavors that really make this breakfast recipe stand out.

Omelet:

This recipe requires only 5 minutes of prep time and your cook time will only be 10 minutes

This recipe serves only one person

Ingredients:

- 2 eggs
- 1 tbsp of romesco sauce
- 1 artichoke heart (make sure it's quartered)
- 2 tbsp of kalamata olives (sliced)
- 2 tbsp of tomato (diced)
- 1 tbsp milk
- 1 tsp oil
- 1 tbsp of feta (make sure it's crumbled)

Instructions:

- Step one: Get a skillet and heat the oil in it.
- Step two: Mix your milk and eggs together and then pour in it and make sure it covers the bottom of the pan that your using.
- Step three: Cook until you see that your egg is beginning to set before adding the olives, artichoke, tomato and cheese on half of your egg.
- Step four: Fold the egg over.

- Step five: Cook until the eggs have set which should only take a minute.
- Step six: Remove from head and use the sauce for the top.
- Step seven: Serve.

Nutritional Information:

Your calories are going to be 303.

Your cholesterol is going to be 337 milligrams.

Your total fat is going to be 17.7 grams.

Your sodium is going to be 631 milligrams.

Your protein is going to be 18.2 grams.

Your total carbohydrates are going to be 21.9 grams.

Your sugar is going to be 4.4 grams.

Your fiber is going to be 9.9 grams.

This recipe is a great favorite from the Mediterranean, but it does take a little longer to make. It is worth the time when you taste the amazing flavor that is behind this recipe.

Eggs the Mediterranean way

This recipe will take only five minutes to prep but an hour and 20 minutes is needed to cook

This recipe will serve 6 people

Ingredients:

- 3 oz of feta cheese (make sure it is crumbled)
- 6 eggs (you may use 2 more if you need to but no more than that)
- 1 garlic clove (make sure it is minced)
- 4 yellow onions (make sure they are small and that us halve them before slicing them. you can go up to 5 but no more)
- 1/3 c sun dried tomatoes (make sure they are julienne cut and that they are firmly packed)
- 1 tbsp olive oil (use extra virgin)
- 1 tbsp butter

There are four ingredients that are optional with this recipe so you may decide if you like them or not with your dish.

If you choose you may add a roll to this recipe and for taste you can add pepper (freshly ground), and salt along with some parsley. If you choose the parsley make sure its finely chopped.

Instructions:

- Step one: You will need a cast iron skillet for this recipe. If you don't have one a stainless one will work as long as its stainless steel. Turn your heat to medium and heat the oil and the butter.

- Step two: After the butter melts you can add in your onions. When you do this you need to stir but do it gently. Try to arrange them in an even layer.
- Step three: Reduce your heat. You want the onions to sizzle but just barely.
- Step four: You need to allow your onions to cook in the skillet. You need to make sure that you stir about every 10 minutes. If that is to long then you will need to stir every 5 minutes instead. This process should take an hour and you will know they are done when they look deeply brown and they are soft.
- Step five: Add your tomatoes to the pan before adding your garlic as well.
- Step six: You will need to stir for 3 minutes until it's fragrant.
- Step seven: Make sure that the mixture is evenly layered in your pan.
- Step eight: When you have done this you can crack the eggs over the top. Be careful when you do this.
- Step nine: You should now sprinkle the top with cheese.
- Step ten: Cover the pan with a lid and make sure that the lid is fitting tightly over the pan and then let it cook for a maximum of 15 minutes and a minimum of 10 minutes.
- Step eleven: The egg yolks will change quickly during the last 5 minutes so watch

them carefully, but you should let the eggs cook undisturbed during the 15 minutes.

- Step twelve: Remove from heat and if desired you can serve this on a roll.

Nutritional Information:

Your calories are going to be 183.

Your cholesterol is going to be 181 milligrams.

Your potassium is going to be 386 milligrams.

Your total fat is going to be 5 grams.

Your sodium is going to be 255 milligrams.

Your protein is going to be 9 grams.

Your total carbohydrates are going to be 11 grams.

Your sugar is going to be 6 grams.

Your fiber is going to be 1 gram.

Toast is a simple breakfast that most take for granted. It's slowly been gaining traction throughout the years and thanks to Instagram it's become a healthy staple of fitness gurus all over.

Avocado Toast:

This recipe will take only 5 minutes of prep and only 2 minutes to cook

This recipe serves only one

Ingredients:

- 1 tsp of honey
- 1 slice of bread (toasted)
- 2 strawberries (slice them thinly)
- A single slice of cheese (white cheddar. Cut into thin little chunks)
- ½ of an avocado

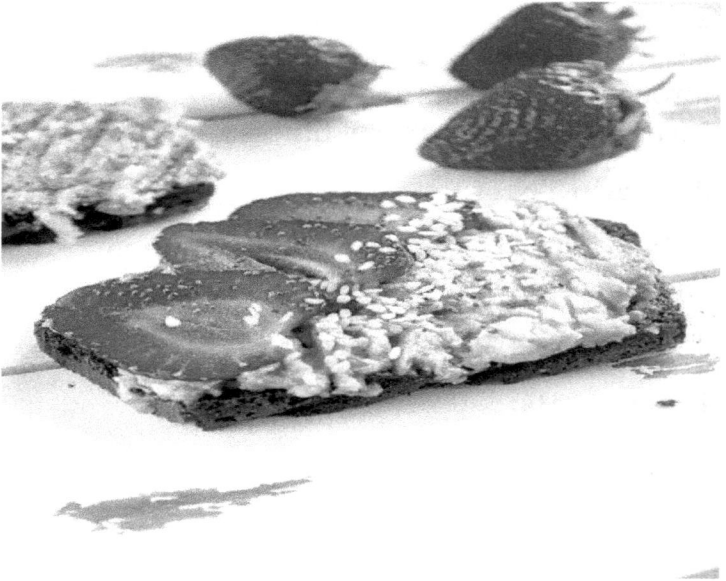

Instructions:

- Step one: Toast the bread.
- Step two: Get a bowl and mash the avocado well.
- Step three: When the bread is finished toasting spread the avocado onto the bread then place the berries and cheese over the top.
- Step four: Drizzle the honey over the top and enjoy your meal.

For another great toast recipe that is easy to make in the morning try this one. It is savory and decadent and should put you in a great mood for starting your day off the right way.

Fig toast:

This recipe takes only 5 minutes of prep time

This recipe serves 2 people **Ingredients:**

- 1 tsp of zest of a lemon
- ½ tbsp of honey
- ¼ c ricotta (make sure its low fat)
- 2 slices of bread (go for gluten free or whole grain for this recipe)
- 4 figs (sliced)
- ½ of a fresh lemon (make sure that it is juiced)
- 2 tbsp of pistachio pieces

Instructions:

- Step one: Toast your bread in your toaster.
- Step two: In a bowl whip your juice, honey, and ricotta together until it is smooth.
- Step three: Spread the mixture onto the toast and then place the figs on top.
- Step four: Sprinkle the pieces of pistachio on top of the toast and then do the same with the zest of the lemon.

Nutritional Information:

This is bases on ½ of the recipe

Your calories are going to be 193.

Your total fat is going to be 6.7 grams.

Your protein is going to be 9 grams.

Your total carbohydrates are going to be 32.3 grams.

Your sugar is going to be 9.3 grams.

Your fiber is going to be 8.1 grams.

Chapter three: Lunch Recipes

Lunch is an important part of your eating as well. People tend to start losing energy around midday which is why some cultures actually eat their biggest meal during midday instead of in the evening. They do this because you not only have enough time to burn it off so you're not gaining weight, but you have the ability to stay energized until you're ready to go to sleep. Other cultures think that eating a small lunch will send a short burst of energy to your system although many studies are still debating this. whichever way you like to eat your lunch you know that you need to be able to make sure that you are getting a variety of recipes that you will actually be able to make use of.

When you're working, thinking about your family's lunches or trying to get some energy to get you through the day, you will need a good meal to get you through it. The work force and jobs that we have today, or school schedules make it practically impossible to get in a good meal and if you're lucky enough that you can, you only have 20 minutes to actually consume it. This means that you need recipes that are quick and easy while making sure that you don't reach for the processed food. With lunch, you need to make sure that you have a recipe that isn't going to take a long time to make and isn't overly complicated.

This chapter offers just what you need. We have great recipes that are mouthwateringly tasty, and some take less than ten minutes to make. This means no matter what you've got going on, you will be able to make sure that your making the healthiest choice possible for your body. With this particular diet, you really have to remember that you need to avoid processed foods and lunch is usually the time when most people reach for fast food and packaged items. You need to avoid doing this otherwise you won't be able to utilize this diet the way you want to. By making the right choices your going to help your body begin to get healthier.

The first recipe that we have is for a chicken wrap. The Mediterranean diet focuses mostly on fish but as long as you're not consuming red meat your allowed to eat other meat. Just not as much. This calls for cooked chicken, so you'll need to do that first. This is the reason it's not in the prep or cook time.

Chicken wrap

This recipe takes 10 minutes of prep time.

This recipe serves 3 people.

Ingredients:

- 3 tortillas (you need to make sure that they are whole wheat)
- ½ of a cup of hummus (feel free to use whatever kind you want but be aware that if you do it's going to change all of your nutritional information, so you will have to recalculate it)
- 1 c of cooked chicken (you may use cubed or shredded chicken)

Instructions:

- Step one: Combine both your hummus and chicken in a bowl.
- Step two: Place on a tortilla and fold to make the wrap.
- Step three: Serve and enjoy

Nutritional information

The serving size is based off of a single tortilla and a half a cup of chicken

Your calories are going to be 225.

Your cholesterol is going to be 40 milligrams.

Your potassium is going to be 214 milligrams.

Your total fat is going to be 8 grams.

Your sodium is going to be 370 milligrams.

Your protein is going to be 21 grams.

Your total carbohydrates are going to be 20 grams.

Your sugar is going to be 1 gram.

Your fiber is going to be 4 grams.

Barley is a good thing for the body and its healthy for you, so this next recipe is for Mediterranean Barley. To stay true to Mediterranean recipes this one will be interesting for you to try for yourself.

Mediterranean Barley

This recipe takes 10 minutes of prep time while the cooking time for this recipe will be around 25 minutes. This is because of the time needed to cook the barley.

This serves 4 people

Ingredients:

- 3 tbsp sun dried tomatoes (make sure that they are packed without any oil and be sure that they are finely chopped)
- 2 tbsp lemon juice (make sure that its fresh)
- 1 c of arugula leaves (make sure that they are packed)
- 1 can of chickpeas (make sure that the can says no salt added. Also, be sure to rinse them and drain them)
- 2 tbsp of olive oil (extra virgin)
- 1 c of pearl barley (uncooked because your going to cook it)
- ½ tsp of red pepper (crushed)
- 2 tbsp of pistachios (chopped)
- 1 c of red bell pepper (chopped finely)

Instructions:

- Step one: Read the barley package and cook the way it says to. Do not put in any salt. For this recipe we are omitting salt.
- Step two: Combine your tomatoes, chickpeas, arugula, barley, and bell pepper in a bowl.
- Step three: Combine your oil, crushed pepper, and lemon juice and then stir.
- Step four: You need to toss the mixture from step two but first you need to drizzle the mixture from step three over the mixture from step two.
- Step five: Toss the mixture to make sure it has been covered.
- Step six: You will now need to sprinkle the top with the pistachios and enjoy the flavor.

Nutritional information:

Serving size is based upon 1 ¼ cups of the barley mixture and 1 and ½ tsp of the pistachios

Your calories are going to be 359.

Your cholesterol is going to be 0 milligrams.

Your potassium is going to be 514 milligrams.

Your total fat is going to be 10 grams.

Your sodium is going to be 852 milligrams.

Your protein is going to be 11 grams.

Your total carbohydrates are going to be 61 grams.

Your sugar is going to be 3 grams.

Your fiber is going to be 14 grams.

This recipe is good for vitamin C as well as potassium.

Our next lunch recipe is pretty visually and tastes great. Most people think that peppers are a hard thing to make but in fact they are very easy. Another thing that may be helpful to know is that peppers aren't always as hot as people think either. This recipe packs a good punch for flavor and will make you excited for your lunch.

Stuffed Peppers

This recipe is going to require 10 minutes of prep time but a half hour (or 30 minutes) for cook time

This recipe will serve four people

Ingredients:

- 1 juiced lime
- 2 tbsp of olive oil
- 1 c of red lentils (uncooked)
- 1/3 c of cilantro (chopped)
- 2 tsp of cumin (ground)
- 4 bell peppers (use medium ones. The great thing about this recipe is that you can use any color you want which lets you get creative)
- ½ of a jalapeno (diced)
- ½ c of chickpeas (they will be canned and need to be rinsed and then drained)
- 1 garlic clove (minced. If you would like to go up to using 2 that's fine as well)
- ½ of an avocado (use a small one and make sure it's diced)

- ½ c of kidney beans (they will be canned and need to be rinsed and then drained)
- ½ c of onion (red)
- 1/3 c of parsley (chopped)
- 2/3 c of tomatoes (heirloom and make sure you diced)
- There are a couple of optional items here including salt and pepper for tasting. If you use them use sea salt. You can also add a half tsp of sumac (ground).

Instructions:

- Step one: Take your peppers and take off of the top. You will need to scoop out the white pulp and scoop out the seeds as well.
- Step two: Set aside.
- Step three: Follow the directions on the package and cook your lentils. They should cook about a half an hour and you will need to add at least a cup of water.
- Step four: In a bowl add in everything except your avocados.
- Step five: You will need to toss everything in the bowl until it is combined.
- Step six: Now you need to scoop that mixture into the bell peppers you set aside.
- Step seven: Place the avocado on top and you have a colorful lunch!

Nutritional information:

This is based off of a single cup

Your calories are going to be 389.

Your cholesterol is going to be 0miligrams.

Your potassium is going to be 1110 milligrams.

Your total fat is going to be 12 grams.

Your sodium is going to be 185 milligrams .

Your protein is going to be 19 grams.

Your total carbohydrates are going to be 54 grams.

Your sugar is going to be 9 gram.

Your fiber is going to be 23 grams.

This recipe is for a simple salad. Salads are usually boring but not here. This one is quick and can be taken anywhere. This salad is chocked full of flavor and vegetables that make this super healthy as well. For a bonus, the tuna and eggs add a nice protein kick as well.

Salad

This recipe takes 12 minutes of prep time

This recipe can serve 2 people

Ingredients:

For the salad:

- 1 tuna can (make it a small can and drain it)
- 8 radishes (go for the French breakfast variety)
- 12 olives (mix black and green)
- 1 bell pepper (make it yellow and then seed it and vein it. Once you have done this slice it thinly)
- 1 onion (make it a small red one and be sure to peel it before slicing it. When you do this slice it in rounds)
- 1 tbsp capers
- 2 fennel bulbs (small ones and trim them before slicing them lengthwise and thinly)
- 2 eggs (hard cooked and quartered)

For the dressing:

- 1 tsp fennel greens (chopped)
- 4 tbsp of olive oil
- 1 tsp of zest of a lemon
- 1 tbsp lemon juice (fresh)
- If you like you may use salt and pepper to taste.

Instructions:

For the dressing:

- Step one: Grab a bowl and combine your oil and juice along with the zest.
- Step two: Make sure that you whisk it until it is smooth.
- Step three: Once you have completed this you will stir in the fennel greens.

For the salad:

- Step one: Take a large plate and begin to arrange your pepper slices that you made and place the fennel slices on top of them.
- Step two: Arrange the radishes as well on the edge but place them scarlet ends out.
- Step three: Arrange the olives around the radishes upon the edge.
- Step four: After you've done this arrange the eggs in twos or threes and place the tuna in a mound in the center.
- Step five: Place the capers on top of the tuna.

- Step six: Set the onions around the salad.
- Step seven: Drizzle the dressing over the top and you're ready to eat.

Nutritional information:

Your calories are going to be 276.

Your total fat is going to be 21 grams.

Your sodium is going to be 505 milligrams.

Your protein is going to be 15 grams.

Your total carbohydrates are going to be 9 grams.

Your fiber is going to be 2 grams.

The Mediterranean diet is influenced by Greek food and this recipe is for a great pizza that is perfect for lunch or dinner. The reason was placing it here is that it only takes about 10 minutes to make.

Pizza from Greece:

This recipe requires a prep time of 5

minutes This recipe will serve a single

person only **Ingredients:**

- 5 kalamata olives (you will need to pit them and halve them)
- 1 slice of pizza crust (it needs to be ready made)
- 5 grape tomatoes (halve them)
- 1 tbsp cheese (use feta chees and make sure that you get crumbled)
- 2 tbsp of red peppers (roasted peppers make sure you drain them)

Instructions:

- Step one: Preheat your oven to 375 exactly.
- Step two: Place your ingredients on top of the pizza in any order that you would like.
- Step three: Bake your pizza for a maximum of 7 minutes. your cheese should be melted.

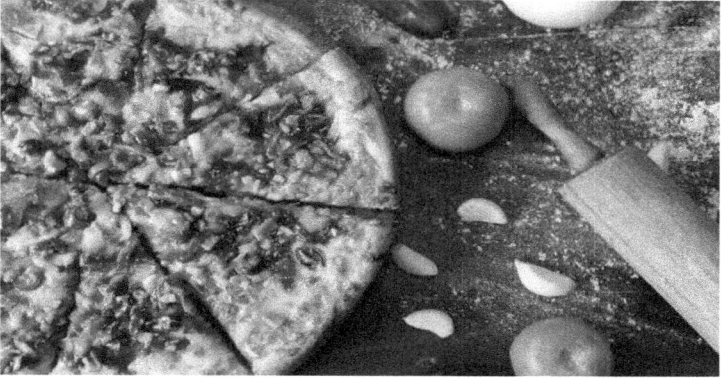

Nutritional information:

Your calories are going to be 260.

Your total fat is going to be 5 grams.

Your sodium is going to be 808 milligrams.

Your protein is going to be 8 grams.

Your total carbohydrates are going to be 47 grams.

Your fiber is going to be 2 grams.

Wraps are a great lunch as well and they are a perfect way to get a serving of vegetables in or another serving of fiber. You'll find that you need to get your nutrition in with each meal, so this is a good way to do it.

Tuna Wrap:

This recipe takes 20 minutes of prep

time This recipe serves 4 people

Ingredients:

- 2 c arugula (use baby version)
- 1 can tuna (use white tuna and make sure it's packed in water not oil. Drain it also)
- 2 tbsp onion (red and chopped)
- 4 wraps (be sure to use omega 3 enriched wraps that are whole wheat)
- 2 tbsp yogurt (use Greek style and make sure its fat free)
- ½ c celery (chopped)
- 1 tbsp of fresh basil (chopped)
- ½ c of white beans (canned. Be sure to rinse and drain them as well.)
- 8 tsp tapenade (a tapenade is an olive spread. Make sure to buy it prepared)
- ¼ tsp of zest from a lemon
- 1 tsp of juice from a lemon

Instructions:

- Step one: In a bowl you will need to stir your zest, juice, yogurt and basil.
- Step two: After you've completed this you will need to stir in your onion, tuna, arugula and celery as well.
- Step three: Place ½ tbsp of the tapenade over each wrap and top with the mixture you made and then roll to make a wrap.

Nutritional Information:

Your calories are going to be 224.

Your total fat is going to be 7 grams.

Your sodium is going to be 682 milligrams.

Your protein is going to be 21 grams.

Your total carbohydrates are going to be 24 grams.

Your fiber is going to be 7 grams.

Chapter four: Snack Recipes

Snacks are a big part of this diet as well because they keep your hunger down and help make sure that you're not overeating. In the meal plan towards the end of the book you will see that your allotted two snacks each day. The snacks of course won't be as big as a meal, but they will help give you energy to keep you going throughout even the busiest day. Snacks are also important if your someone who works out a lot and is a fitness inclined person. Even with these recipes and diet you will still need to exercise as well. This means you will need some protein and nutrients after your workout.

Like the other sections most of these recipes make decent amounts of servings so this will cut down on the cooking for you because you have enough leftover for at least one more meal and in some cases two or three. The difference between the recipes in this book and others is that these are healthy. When most people think of snacking, they think of cookies and candy. That is how people become overweight and obese. When that happens your knees, mind, organs and liver can suffer. Not only that your physical and mental state can deteriorate as well.

Choosing healthy options is the best way to counter this. Another tip for snacking is to make sure you're not in front of a television or if you're bored. Studies have shown that this causes people to snack more on junk food and to eat more than they want. An even better tip is to make sure that your getting a full night sleep or you'll snack all night which is what you don't want. Instead try one of these recipes on for size and see how great they taste.

Hummus is a great compliment to vegetables and bread or crackers and in the meal plan we have outlined for you; you will see hummus appear a few times in the snack section. What better way to try it than to make it yourself?

Hummus:

This recipe takes 10 minutes of prep time

This recipe will serve 14 people

Ingredients:

- Lemon juice from 2 lemons
- Red pepper (ground)
- 5 tsp of tahini
- 3 garlic cloves (minced)
- 1 can of chickpeas (be sure to rinse them and drain them)
- Soy sauce (reduced sodium)
- 1 tbsp olive oil (extra virgin)
- 1/3 c yogurt (make it plain and nonfat)
- ¼ c parsley (make sure its packed finely and fresh. Then mince it)
- ¼ c of scallions (minced)

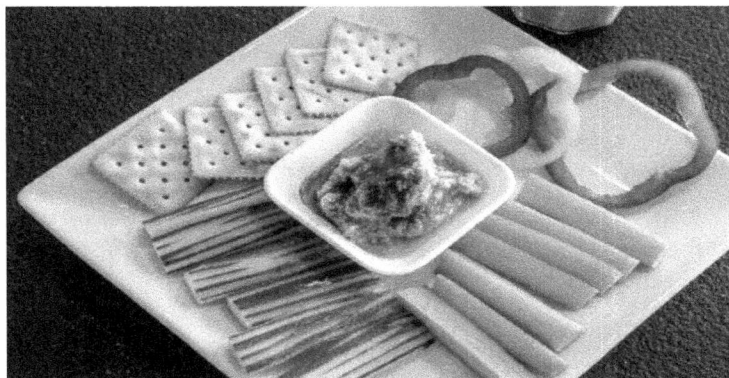

Instructions:

- Step one: Using a food processor and blend the chickpeas until they are smooth.
- Step two: Add your other ingredients to the processor as well (except the red pepper) and blend once more until smooth.
- Step three: Place in a bowl and place red pepper on top.
- Step four: Be sure to serve at room temperature.

Nutritional information:

This is based per serving

Your calories are going to be 61.

Your total fat is going to be 2 grams.

Your sodium is going to be 97 milligrams.

Your protein is going to be 2 grams.

Your total carbohydrates are going to be 9 grams.

Your fiber is going to be 2 grams.

Pudding can make a good snack or dessert but this one is going to be listed as a snack because of the nuts that you will find in it.

Pumpkin pudding:

This recipe takes 15 minutes of prep time

This recipe serves 4 people

Ingredients:

For the pudding:

- ¼ c maple syrup
- 1 c of pumpkin puree
- 2 tsp of pumpkin spice
- ½ c of chia seeds
- 1 ¼ c of any milk you choose

If desired, you may use the following for toppings:

Blueberries, almonds, and sunflower seeds. If you choose to use these the amount will be a fourth of a cup each.

Instructions:

- Step one: Place all the ingredients into a bowl and mix.
- Step two: Let it stand for 15 minutes. You can also put it in the refrigerator overnight if you like.
- Step three: Serve with toppings if desired.

Nutritional information:

This is based per serving

Your calories are going to be 189.

Your cholesterol is going to be 6 milligrams.

Your potassium is going to be 311 milligrams.

Your total fat is going to be 7.6 grams.

Your sodium is going to be 42 milligrams .

Your protein is going to be 5.9 grams.

Your total carbohydrates are going to be 27 grams.

Your sugar is going to be 18.5 grams.

Your fiber is going to be 4.4 grams.

Cucumbers are a really healthy snack and as we've mentioned hummus is a great snack to utilize as well. For this snack, were going to combine the two.

Cucumbers with hummus:

This recipe takes ten minutes of prep time and 5 minutes of cook time

This recipe serves 6

Ingredients:

- 5 cucumbers (medium)
- 1 c carrot (sliced)
- 2 green onions (use large ones and have them chopped)
- 4 garlic cloves (peeled)
- ½ tsp paprika
- ½ c of tahini
- ¼ c of lemon juice (add a tbsp to this and make sure the juice is fresh)
- 15 oz of navy beans (canned and you will need to drain them and then rinse them)

Instructions:

- Step one: You will need to have a steamer and use it to steam the garlic cloves (they should be whole) and carrots for 5 minutes in simmering water.
- Step two: Take it off the steamer and place it in a food processor.
- Step three: Add the beans and blend till smooth.
- Step four: Add in your tahini and blend till smooth as well.
- Step five: Drizzle the lemon in and add paprika before mixing.
- Step six: Place in a bowl.
- Step seven: After washing the cucumbers cut them to your preference and then enjoy your snack.

- Step eight: If desired you may use the onions as a garnish or for flavor.

Nutritional Information:

This is based on half a cucumber and 3 tbsp of hummus

Your calories are going to be 234.

Your total fat is going to be 10 grams.

Your sodium is going to be 290 milligrams.

Your protein is going to be 11 grams.

Your total carbohydrates are going to be 22 grams.

Your sugar is going to be 6 grams.

Your fiber is going to be 8 grams.

Grapefruit is also a good fruit for a snack and were pairing it with a yogurt sauce this time for a more flavorful and authentic feel.

Grapefruit Time:

This recipe requires 10 minutes of prep time and 5 minutes of cook time

This recipe serves 4 people

Ingredients:

- 1 tbsp of honey (make sure its raw)
- 2 grapefruits (make sure they are large)
- 2 tbsp of pine nuts (make sure they are unsalted)
- A single pomegranate (make sure it is large)
- ¼ c of yogurt (make sure its Greek and nonfat. Also, be sure that it is plain)

Instructions:

- Step one: Take a bowl and fill it with cool water.
- Step two: Take the pomegranate and take the seeds out.
- Step three: You will need to add arils to the bowl.
- Step four: You will need to make sure that the grapefruits are peeled and then cut them into segments.
- Step five: Discard the pith and the peel.
- Step six: When this is completed you can add the grapefruit to the bowl with the arils from the pomegranate.
- Step seven: Carefully and gently toss to make sure that the items combine.
- Step eight: In a separate bowl stir the honey and yogurt together until its smooth.
- Step nine: Take a skillet and put it on a medium heat.

- Step ten: Add in the nuts and toast them. This process is going to take 3 minutes maximum. During this process you will need to shake the skillet. You will also need to make sure that they are fragrant and golden.
- Step eleven: Remove from heat.
- Step twelve: Place the suave over the top of everything and then place the nuts on top.
- Step thirteen: Enjoy your snack.

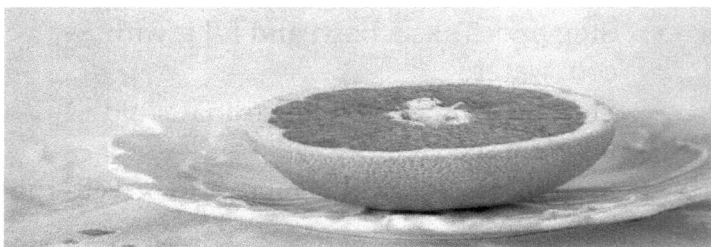

Nutritional Information:

Serving is based on 1 tbsp of sauce, ¼ c of the arils, ½ a grapefruit and ½ a tbsp of the nuts

Your calories are going to be 125.

Your total fat is going to be 2 grams.

Your sodium is going to be 8 milligrams.

Your protein is going to be 4 grams.

Your total carbohydrates are going to be 26 grams.

Your sugar is going to be 23grams.

Your fiber is going to be 2 grams.

Skewers are fun at dinner or at snack time. This one is fun for adults and children a like and they are simple and easy to make.

Fruit and Veggie Skewers:

This recipe requires only 5 minutes of prep

time This will serve one person **Ingredients:**

- ¼ mozzarella balls (use baby mozzarella)
- 1 peach (medium and make it sliced)
- ½ c tomatoes (cherry kind)
- 4 basil leaves (fresh)

Instructions:

- Step one: Get a wooden skewer.
- Step two: Arrange your ingredients on the skewer however you like
- Step three: repeat twice more for a total of three.

Nutritional Information:

This is based on three skewers

Your calories are going to be 143.

Your cholesterol is going to be 20 milligrams.

Your potassium is going to be 467 milligrams.

Your total fat is going to be 6 grams.

Your sodium is going to be 90 milligrams.

Your protein is going to be 7 grams.

Your total carbohydrates are going to be 17 grams.

Your sugar is going to be 14 grams.

Your fiber is going to be 3 grams.

This recipe is great for vitamin A and C because it is over 30 percent of your daily value in vitamin C and over 25 percent in your vitamin A.

If you are a meal prepper or need to reach for something quick, then this is perfect for you. With a great Mediterranean feel, this is great for the diet and will perk you right up.

Snack Pack Attack:

This recipe takes only 5 minutes to

prep It serves one person

Ingredients:

- 6 olives (make sure that they are oil cured)
- 10 tomatoes (make sure they are the cherry kind)
- 1 slice of bread (use whole wheat bread and try to get a crusty version. Cut into little pieces)
- ¼ oz of cheese (make sure it's aged and sliced)

Instructions:

- Step one: Place the items on a plate in whatever decorative fashion that you wish.

Nutritional information:

Your calories are going to be 197.

Your cholesterol is going to be 5 milligrams.

Your potassium is going to be 475 milligrams.

Your total fat is going to be 9 grams.

Your sodium is going to be 674 milligrams.

Your protein is going to be 7 grams.

Your total carbohydrates are going to be 22 grams.

Your sugar is going to be 6 grams.

Your fiber is going to be 4 grams.

This recipe is great for vitamin A and C. This recipe is over 35 percent of your daily value of vitamin C and over 25 percent of your vitamin A.

Chapter five: Dinner Recipes

Dinner is important for anyone. You need to make sure that you have one that is healthy and can fill you without making you overeat unnecessarily. A healthy dinner can make your body feel good and help you sleep. Sleep is an important part of being healthy and the foods you eat affect how you sleep. Since dinner is the last meal you'll be eating, this is especially important. It can also keep those hunger pangs at bay. The problem with most diets is that people think that they can only eat certain things and they can't indulge in their favorite meals. This means they end up having multiple cheat days or completely wrecking all of their hard work because they are so hungry. With these recipes you won't have to worry about that because we've got all your bases covered. Other benefits of a good healthy meal are that it helps relax your mind as well as your body.

Eating with family or friends also cultivates a strong sense of self as well as a sense of family love and community. It also opens you to new experiences and flavors that you may not have experienced before. This diet is a great way to open yourself up to cooking and learning new dishes, but it also lets you see that this diet has a lot of differences than others. You don't have to give up your favorite foods like pizza. You just have to be more mindful about what goes in it.

There are many ways that you can adopt a new diet or lifestyle, you just need to learn the ins and outs of how to do it.

In this section we will be giving some great recipes for dinners that you can eat either alone or with family and they are a tasty but healthy alternative to the way you eat now. Another plus for this section is that the meals don't take to long to prepare and the ones that do its mostly oven time meaning that you can still do other things while your cooking and you don't have to worry about being glued to the kitchen.

The first recipe was going to be showing you is pizza. Pizza is a favorite of almost anyone, but it can rack up the calories and it can rack up your chances to gain weight because of the grease and processed foods that go into pizza. The processed meats alone can add unnecessary issues. This pizza, however, is totally different. The crust is cauliflower which is so much healthier for you and the sauce? Yogurt. Enjoy a great new twist on an old favorite.

Pizza

The prep time you will need for this recipe is 20 minutes while the cook time is an hour

This will serve 4 people

Ingredients:

Crust:

- 2 egg whites (large)
- 1 1/3 c and an additional 4 tbsp of cheese (parmesan divide it and grate it)
- 1 tsp of Italian seasoning
- 1 tbsp and an additional 1 tsp of garlic (minced)
- 12 c of cauliflower (you will need to cut this int florets)

Sauce:

- 1 tbsp of olive oil
- ½ c of fresh basil (you will need to make sure that this is roughly chopped and that its fresh. Also, be sure to pack it firmly)
- ½ c of yogurt (it needs to be Greek and it needs to be nonfat. Go for plain.)
- 2 tsp of garlic (minced)

Topping:

- ½ c cheese (parmesan and be sure to grate it)
- Roma tomatoes (use three inch ones and slice them a half inch thick)
- ½ tbsp of olive oil
- 1 zucchini (sliced and use a small one)
- If you desire, you may also have basil for a garnish if you do this be sure that it's fresh

Instructions:

- Step one: You will need to preheat your oven to 400 degrees exactly.
- Step two: You will need to line a pizza pan (use parchment paper).
- Step three: Get a food processor and use it to process the cauliflower. You will need to do this until it is at the texture of rice.
- Step four: You will need to put your cauliflower into a bowl and place it in the microwave for no more than 7 minutes.

- Step five: You need to stir and then microwave for another 7 minutes.
- Step six: Let the cauliflower cool. It shouldn't be more than 15 minutes.
- Step seven: Place the cauliflower onto a kitchen towel.
- Step eight: Ring out all of the moisture. Make sure it is all gone. If it's not it will affect the crust.
- Step nine: Put the cauliflower back into your bowl and then add in the seasoning and the garlic.
- Step ten: Add in the cheese.
- Step eleven: Stir all the ingredients until everything is combined in the bowl.
- Step twelve: Add in your eggs whites and stir again until it's combined again.
- Step thirteen: Turn your cauliflower into 4 separate balls and then place on the pizza pan. Be sure to spread them out and then leave yourself a ridge for the crust of the pizza.
- Step fourteen: Now you need to bake it until its brown. This will take a half hour (30 minutes)
- Step fifteen: Place your remaining garlic, basil and yogurt in the processes or and make sure you make it creamy.
- Step sixteen: You will also need to stream in the olive oil while the food processor is on and make sure that its mixed well.

- Step seventeen: Set it aside.
- Step eighteen: Preheat your grill to a heat that is medium high.
- Step nineteen: Combine your remaining olive oil and tomato along with the zucchini in a bowl.
- Step twenty: Grill until it has charred. This will take 3 minutes.
- Step twenty one: Set aside but make sure that you leave the grill on because you will need it once more.
- Step twenty two: When your pizza is done remove it from the oven and then preheat your broiler.
- Step twenty three: Heat for 3 minutes.
- Step twenty four: Use part of the cheese and then place on top of the pizza.
- Step twenty five: You need to broil for 3 minutes until it's golden brown.
- Step twenty six: Spread the sauce on the pizzas and then top with the veggies and sprinkle the remaining cheese over the top.
- Step twenty seven: Place the pizzas on the grill and cook for 3 minutes. This will melt the cheese.
- Step twenty eight: Serve immediately.

Nutritional information:

This is based on one serving.

Your calories are going to be 331.

Your cholesterol is going to be 26.5 milligrams.

Your total fat is going to be 16.3 grams.

Your sodium is going to be 1552.2 milligrams.

Your protein is going to be 27 grams.

Your total carbohydrates are going to be 23.7 grams.

Your sugar is going to be 10.1 grams.

As a side note this recipe is great for vitamin C.

Are you a fan of gyros? We have a great recipe for them that will make your mouth water. It doesn't take to much time in under thirty minutes, but the effort is well worth it because it's not only quick it's easy to make and it is kid friendly as well if you have children which makes it even better.

Gyro

This recipe will take just 10 minutes of prep time but 16 minutes to cook.

This recipe will serve 4 people

Ingredients:

For the meatball:

- 1 tsp oregano
- 1 pound of ground turkey
- 2 tbsp olive oil
- 1 c of spinach (make sure it's fresh and chopped)
- 2 cloves of garlic (minced)
- ¼ c red onion (red onion and diced finely)

Sauce:

- 1 c of cucumber (diced)
- 1 c of tomato (diced)
- ½ tsp of garlic powder
- 2 tbsp of lemon juice
- 4 flatbreads (make sure they are whole wheat)

- ¼ c of cucumber (grated)
- ½ c onion (red onion and make sure to thinly slice it)
- ½ yogurt (make sure that its Greek and plain)
- ½ dill (dry)

Instructions:

- Step one: Get a large bowl.
- Step two: Add the spinach, onion, garlic, oregano, and turkey.
- Step three: Mix the ingredients together and make balls (make sure they stick together).
- Step four: Turn heat to medium high and heat your skillet.
- Step five: Add your olive oil to your pan.
- Step six: Add the meatballs to the pan and cook each side of the meatball for 3 minutes. If you need an additional minute that's fine but you shouldn't need more than 4.
- Step six: When all sides have been completely browned, then you can remove them from the pan and then place to the side.
- Step seven: Add dill, grated cucumber, lemon juice, and yogurt along with the garlic powder into a bowl.
- Step eight: Mix it all together until it has combined well.

- Step nine: To assemble your dish, take a flatbread and add 2 meatballs or 3 if they fit, and the tomato, cucumber, and onion.
- Step ten: Top your gyro with sauce.
- Step eleven: Serve and enjoy

Nutritional information:

The serving for this recipe is based on the meatballs and flatbread.

Your calories are going to be 429.

Your cholesterol is going to be 91 milligrams.

Your total fat is going to be 19 grams.

Your sodium is going to be 630 milligrams.

Your protein is going to be 28 grams.

Your total carbohydrates are going to be 38 grams.

Your sugar is going to be 4 grams.

Our next recipe is for a simple tuna salad with a nice twist. Tuna salad is packed with protein and this one has a great zest that tastes great but doesn't take much time. This is great for beginners and has enough for leftovers as well.

Tuna Salad

This recipe takes about 10 minutes of prep time

This recipe serves 6 people

Ingredients:

- 2 cans of tuna (make sure that it's the chunk light tuna in water not oil. You will also need to drain it well)
- ½ of an onion (red and chopped finely)
- ½ of a bunch of mint (chopped finely)
- 2 tomatoes (roam and chopped)
- 1 tbsp of olive oil
- 2 cans of chickpeas (rinse them and chop them roughly)
- 1 garlic clove (minced)
- 1 bunch flat parsley leaf (chopped finely)
- ½ tsp of zest of a lemon
- 3 tbsp of lemon juice

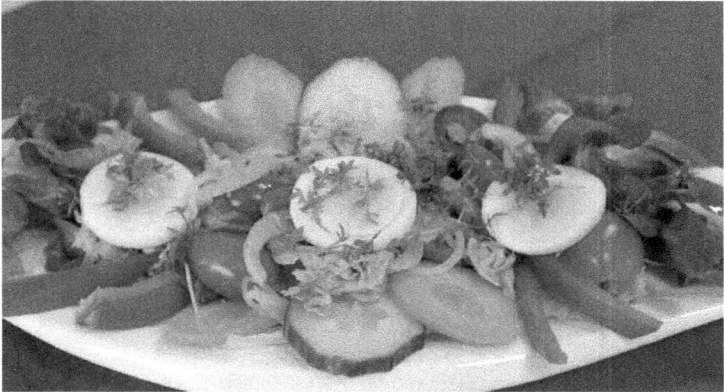

Instructions:

- Step one: Get a large bowl.
- Step two: Combine all of your ingredients in the bowl but make sure that you add the tuna in last.
- Step three: Serve and enjoy.

Nutritional Information:

The serving size is based on a half cup

Your calories are going to be 280.

Your total fat is going to be 5.7 grams.

Your protein is going to be 21.4 grams.

Your total carbohydrates are going to be 36 grams.

Your sugar is going to be 1 gram.

As we have mentioned this diet is big on the fish, so the next recipe is for salmon. This is very easy, and it is also very fresh. It has a good flavor instead of just being plain. It's great if you have guests as well and it doesn't take much to make it at all.

Baked Salmon

This recipe takes 10 minutes of prep time while taking 10 minutes to cook

This recipe will serve 4 people

Ingredients:

- 4 wedges of lemon
- 1 ½ tbsp dill (fresh and chopped finely)
- 4 fillets of salmon (make sure that they are an inch thick but not more)
- If you like you can season with kosher salt and fresh black pepper

Instructions:

- Step one: You will need to preheat your oven to 350 exactly
- Step two: Coat a baking sheet with cooking spray
- Step three: Place your fish on the sheet
- Step four: Make sure to coat your fish lightly with the cooking spray

- Step five: You will now sprinkle your fish with the seasonings if your choosing to use it and the dill as well.
- Step six: Bake the fish for 10 minutes (you will know when it's done when the fish flakes easily. You can test this with a fork).
- Step seven: You can use the lemon wedges when your serving the dish.
- Step eight: Enjoy your meal.

Nutritional information:

Serving size is based on a single lemon wedge with a single fillet

Your calories are going to be 251.

Your cholesterol is going to be 94 milligrams.

Your potassium is going to be 845 milligrams.

Your total fat is going to be 12 grams.

Your sodium is going to be 215 milligrams.

Your protein is going to be 34 grams.

Your total carbohydrates are going to be 1 gram.

Your sugar is going to be 0 grams.

Your fiber is going to be 0 grams.

The next recipe we have can work for lunch or dinner, but we've chosen to put it in the dinner section because it takes over a half an hour to cook. This Mediterranean cod is great for protein, but it's also packed with flavor that lets you know this is one tasty diet.

Mediterranean Cod

This recipe takes 15 minutes of prep time and 45 minutes to cook

This recipe serves 4 people

Ingredients:

- 2 garlic cloves (minced)
- 2 red bell peppers (you need to have them trimmed before halving them and seeding them)
- 1 tsp of olive oil (make sure that it's divided)
- 10 kalamata olives (pitted and minced)
- 2 tbsp lemon juice (fresh)
- ¾ c flat leaf parsley (packed and fresh and then mince it)
- ½ tsp of zest of a lemon
- If desired, you can season with sea salt and black pepper (ground)
- 4 cod fillets (skinless and boneless make sure that they are 5 ounces)
- 2 c of spinach (use baby spinach)

Salad:

Ingredients:

- 10 kalamata olives (pitted and chopped)
- 1 ½ c of grape tomatoes (chopped)
- 2 tsp of olive oil
- 1 garlic clove (minced)
- 1 tbsp of oregano (dry)
- 1 can chickpeas (use a can that is BPA free and make sure that it is unsalted. Drain them before rinsing them and make sure you pat them dry)
- ½ of a red onion (chopped)
- ½ c flat leaf parsley (packed and freshly make sure that you mince it and divide it)
- 1 ½ tsp of zest from a lemon
- ¼ c lemon juice (fresh)
- ¼ cup feta cheese (use crumbled)

Instructions:

- Step one: You will need to preheat your oven to exactly 350 degrees.
- Step two: Using foil line a baking sheet.
- Step three: Place 2 garlic cloves, 10 olives, and 2 tsp of the lemon juice in a small bowl and combine them.
- Step four: Set it aside.
- Step five: On the baking sheet place your bell peppers on it. You need to make sure

that the skin is the down side and it should be open on top.

- Step six: Be sure to brush the tops of the peppers with ¼ of a tsp of oil. For this step be sure that your making sure the oil is being divided evenly.
- Step seven: You will then need to make sure that you top each of the halves with ½ a cup of the spinach.
- Step eight: After completing this add one cod fillet to the halves.
- Step nine: To the olive mix that you set aside before you will need to add the remaining olive oil and then stir.
- Step ten: Spread your mixture over the cod and make sure that it has been divided evenly.
- Step eleven: You should now bake the cod. It will take at least 20 minutes but shouldn't take more than 25. It should flake easily.
- Step twelve: While the cod is baking, we can concentrate on your salad. Get yourself a skillet and heat it to a medium high heat.
- Step thirteen: You should then heat 2 tsp of the oil on the heat.
- Step fourteen: Add your garlic (only one clove) and onion to the skillet and cook for a single minute.

- Step fifteen: Now add in your lemon juice and ¼ a cup of your parsley as well as the chickpeas and a tbsp of water.
- Step sixteen: Cook for 5 but remember to stir it often.
- Step seventeen: Add your tomatoes and 10 chopped olives before cooking again and stirring like you did before. This should take about 8 minutes and you should see the liquid evaporating.
- Step eighteen: You should now stir in the cheese and remaining parsley.
- Step nineteen: Add the zest from the lemon and if you choose to season with pepper, that as well.
- Step twenty: Remove from heat.
- Step twenty one: Being very careful lift the pepper halves off of the baking sheet and place them on plates.
- Step twenty two: Serve the cod with the salad.

Nutritional Information:

The serving size is based on a cod, half a cup of salad, half a bell pepper and a half a cup of spinach.

Your calories are going to be 363.

Your cholesterol is going to be 69 milligrams.

Your total fat is going to be 10 grams.

Your sodium is going to be 455 milligrams.

Your protein is going to be 35 grams.

Your total carbohydrates are going to be 33 grams.

Your sugar is going to be 7 grams.

Your fiber is going to be 8 grams.

This is going to be another good chicken recipe. You will have a lot of vegetables which makes this dish really healthy as well as having good flavor combinations in the food. The prep and cook time are a little longer but it's still a great recipe for beginners because it's easy to make and it works well.

Chicken and Vegetables

The prep time for this recipe takes 15 minutes while the cooking takes 40.

This will serve 4 people

Ingredients:

- 4 chicken thighs (you can choose to use boneless or chicken that still has the bones)
- 3 cloves of garlic (they need to be large and they will need to be minced)
- 4 sage leaves (make sure that they are fresh and that you have chopped them)
- A pound of butternut squash (you should cut the squash into pieces that are small enough to bite)
- 1 lemon (slice it thinly)
- 1 tbsp of apple cider vinegar
- 1 tsp of red pepper (crushed)
- 2 tbsp of balsamic vinegar
- 1 tsp garlic powder
- 1 tsp of paprika (ground)

- A pound of Brussel sprouts (you need to trim them and then halve them)
- ½ onion (medium and chopped)
- 2 tbsp of olive oil
- 1 tsp of fennel seeds
- Pinch of nutmeg (freshly grated is needed)

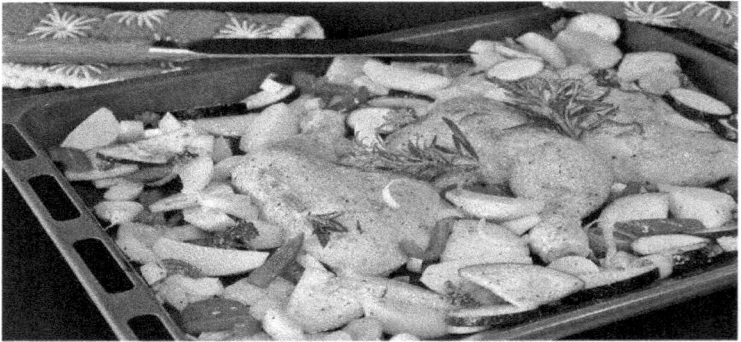

Instructions:

- Step one: You will need to preheat your oven to exactly 450 degrees.
- Step two: You will need to combine your minced garlic, onion, slices of lemon, brussels sprouts, and squash in a bowl.
- Step three: Add in 2 tbsp of the balsamic vinegar and oil along with the nutmeg and toss it. This is going to make it combine.
- Step four: Spread the mixture you've just made onto a baking sheet.
- Step five: Get yourself a bowl.
- Step six: In that bowl you have, add in all of your fennel seeds, garlic powder, red

pepper, apple cider vinegar, paprika, olive oil, and your sage.

- Step seven: This is going to be used as a marinade for the chicken so what your going to do here is use this mixture that you just made to coat your chicken.
- Step eight: Place your chicken on top of the vegetable mix you made before.
- Step nine: Place in the oven and then proceed to bake your dish. This will take a minimum of 30 minutes and a maximum for 40 minutes (by this time the chicken should be cooked completely through, and your veggies should be as well).
- Step ten: Plate your dish when its finished baking and then squeeze juice from the lemon over each plate.

Nutritional Information:

The serving size is based on ¼ of the recipe above

Your calories are going to be 348.

Your cholesterol is going to be 80 milligrams.

Your potassium is going to be 1135 milligrams.

Your total fat is going to be 18 grams.

Your sodium is going to be 680 milligrams.

Your protein is going to be 22 grams.

Your total carbohydrates are going to be 30 grams.

Your sugar is going to be 7 grams.

Your fiber is going to be 8 grams.

This recipe is great for vitamin A and C.

Turkey burgers are also on the rise because people are trying to stay away from certain types of meat. This turkey burger packs on the protein and makes sure that your stomach is completely satisfied.

Turkey burger:

This recipe takes 10 minutes of prep time and about 20 minutes of cook time

This recipe will serve 4 people

Ingredients:

For the burger:

- 1 tbsp of milk
- 1 tbsp of mint (make sure that it is fresh. You will need to chop it)
- ½ c of cheese (use feta and make sure it's crumbled)
- A pound of ground turkey
- 1 tbsp of parsley (make sure its fresh and make sure that you chop it)

For the sauce of the burger:

- 1 tbsp of mint (make sure that it is fresh, and you will need to chop it)
- 1 container of yogurt (use 6 oz and make sure its Greek. Also make sure that it's plain.
- 1 tbsp of lemon juice
- A single clove of garlic (minced)

- A tbsp of parsley (make sure that it is fresh and be sure to chop it up)

Instructions:

- Step one: Wash hands thoroughly before getting a bowl and placing the milk, cheese, mint and parsley, and the turkey in the bowl.
- Step two: Mix with your hands until you see that its thoroughly combined.
- Step three: Make 4 patties with the mixture.
- Step four: If your using a grill you will need to heat it up and if you are using a stove the you need to place a pan (grill pan) over a heat that is medium high.
- Step five: Grill your burgers until they are cooked through. You will be able to tell because the inside will not be pink at all.
- Step six: For the sauce part of the recipe you will need to get another bowl and place all the ingredients on the list inside of it.
- Step seven: Combine the ingredients and make sure they have been done well.
- Step eight: You can place the sauce on the burgers or on the side but now you can enjoy.

Nutritional information:

- This is based off of a single burger
- Your calories will be 204.
- Your protein will be 12 grams.
- Your total carbohydrates will be 0 grams.
- Your total fat will be 12 grams.

Chapter six: Dessert Recipes

Dessert is many people's favorite part of any day, but the problem is most diets don't allow for desserts because of the high sugar content and fat content. It has long since been told to us that desserts will ruin our diet and that we aren't allowed to indulge because it will cause us to gain weight as well. This diet? Dessert is your friend and it's okay to indulge (In moderation of course. You obviously wouldn't be able to eat dessert every day or all day because that would of course be too much).

Dessert doesn't have to be the enemy. What we need to realize about dessert is that if you do it the right way, it can be alright. It's when we indulge in a bad way that leads to unhealthy eating habits, but this can be fixed now with these all new recipes. The recipes we will be having you learn how to make things like pudding which would normally shoot your macros complete out of the zone. With this diet you don't have to worry about that because the recipes stay where you need them to through careful calculations of what it is you need.

Another thing that's helpful is that they don't take long to make so as a beginner it should give you no trouble at all while letting you indulge your sweet tooth in a healthy manner. The deserts on the Mediterranean diet has specific foods that your going to need to cut out so obviously you won't find them here. You will however be able to find that you have sweet taste and healthy options with these wonderful recipes.

Are you a fan of pudding? Many are. If this includes you, then your in luck. This recipe is for a decadent pudding that will have you refusing to share with anyone. A bonus? It has healthy ingredients.

Chocolate pudding:

This recipe only needs 5 minutes of prep time and no cooking time at all

This recipe will serve 4 people

Ingredients:

- 2 tsp of extract of vanilla
- 1/3 c of cacao powder (make sure its raw)
- 2 avocados (make sure that you use large ones and make sure they are chilled)
- ½ c of coconut milk (make sure its full fat)
- 1/3 c of maple syrup

Your toppings are optional but if you'd like it, you can use a little sea salt and hazelnuts. If you use hazelnuts chop them up roughly.

Instructions:

- Step one: Take the avocados and slice them in half. Then you will need to remove the pit.
- Step two: You will now need to scoop the flesh out and put it in a food processor.

- Step three: Add in the rest of the ingredients and make sure you blend until its creamy.
- Step four: Serve with toppings if desired.

Nutritional information:

Serving size is based upon a single cup

Your calories are going to be 295.3.

Your total fat is going to be 20.9 grams.

Your sodium is going to be 10.3 milligrams.

Your protein is going to be 3.4 grams.

Your total carbohydrates are going to be 29.1 grams.

Your sugar is going to be 16.5 grams.

Your fiber is going to be 7.3 grams.

Yogurt bowls are popular in the Mediterranean and in other countries. The difference is how they eat them. In the United States for example, many eat a yogurt bowl for breakfast. In the Mediterranean they like to eat them for a dessert which is why we are placing it here.

Greek yogurt bowl:

This recipe requires 5 minutes of prep time

This recipe will serve 4 people

Ingredients:

- ¼ c of peanut butter (go for natural and be sure that its creamy)
- 4 c of yogurt (make sure it is Greek and that its vanilla)
- ¼ c of flax seed meal
- 1 tsp of nutmeg (for added flavor)
- 2 bananas (Sliced and use medium ones)

Instructions:

- Step one: Because this serves four, you will need four bowls.
- Step two: Split the yogurt into the bowls and top with bananas.
- Step three: Melt the peanut butter in the microwave for a maximum of 40 seconds.
- Step four: Drizzle it over each bowl.
- Step five: Place the nutmeg and flaxseed over the top.

Nutritional information:

This is based per serving

Your calories are going to be 370.

Your cholesterol is going to be 10 milligrams.

Your total fat is going to be 10.6 grams.

Your sodium is going to be 146 milligrams .

Your protein is going to be 22.7 grams.

Your total carbohydrates are going to be 47.7 grams.

Your sugar is going to be 35.8 grams.

Your fiber is going to be 4.7 grams.

You will notice that this recipe is high in sugar. This is because of the sugar that is in the ingredients that are required for this recipe. It is also very carb heavy. Since the Mediterranean diet wants you to stay away from too much sugar, this is going to be something that you indulge in once in awhile not all the time.

Popsicles are another treat, and these ones are from Mediterranean cuisine. This of course fits in with your diet and deserves to be looked at closer.

Popsicles:

This recipe takes ten minutes of prep time and 4 hours of freezing time

This recipe serves 8 people

Ingredients:

- ½ c of milk (go for almond)
- 2 ½ c of berries (use strawberries)

Instructions:

- Step one: Be sure to wash your strawberries under cold water.
- Step two: Rinse all of the strawberries and then remove the hull.
- Step three: Use a blender and blend your ingredients until they are smooth.
- Step four: Put them into molds with sticks and then freeze for 4 hours before consuming.

Nutritional Information:

Your calories are going to be 139.

Your cholesterol is going to be 0 milligrams.

Your potassium is going to be 549.5 milligrams.

Your total fat is going to be 2.3 grams.

Your sodium is going to be 8.3 milligrams .

Your protein is going to be 2.9 grams.

Your total carbohydrates are going to be 31 grams.

Your sugar is going to be 20.6 grams.

Your fiber is going to be 7.5 grams.

Apples are a wonderful dessert and they are a typical Mediterranean dessert. This one is super simple and it's perfect as a sweet treat before you go to bed.

Apple Treat:

This recipe requires 5 minutes of prep time

This recipe will only serve a single person

Ingredients:

- 1/8 tsp cinnamon (for flavor)
- 1 apple (cut it into slices. If you can get it local)
- ½ tsp of honey

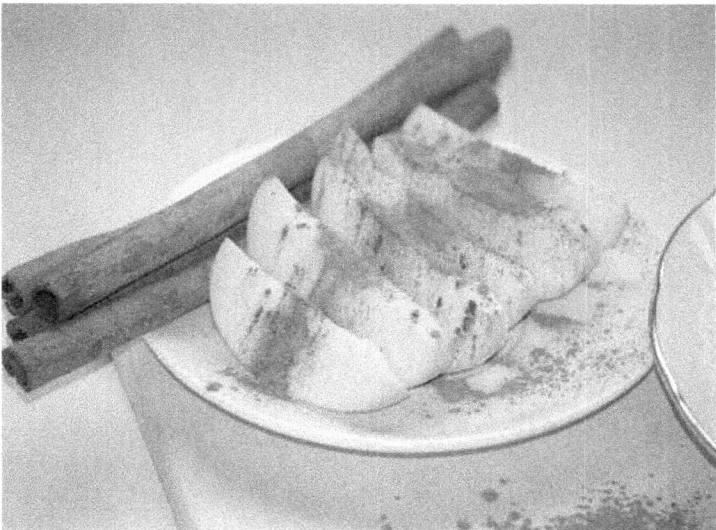

Instructions:

- Step one: Place the apple slices onto a plate.
- Step two: Place the honey and cinnamon over the top of the slices.
- Step three: Enjoy your dish.

Pears are another great Mediterranean desert that tastes amazing. This is another great idea for beginners because it's very easy to master and doesn't have a lot of fuss.

Baked Pears:

This recipe requires 5 minutes of prep time while requiring 25 minutes of cook time

This recipe will serve 4 people

Ingredients:

- ½ c of maple syrup (make sure it's pure)
- 1 tsp of extract of vanilla (make sure it's pure)
- 4 Anjou pears
- ¼ tsp cinnamon (ground)

Instructions:

- Step one: You will need to preheat your oven to 375 degrees exactly.
- Step two: You will need to cut your pears in half.
- Step three: Then you will need to cut a tiny sliver off of the underside of the pear. If you don't they won't sit flat on the baking sheet.
- Step four: Take out the seeds.
- Step five: Place them face up on the sheet.
- Step six: Place the cinnamon on top.

- Step seven: Mix the extract and syrup together and then spread it over the pears. Save a few tbsp for after the baking.
- Step eight: Bake. This will take about 25 minutes. you will know when they are done when they are browned at the edges and soft.
- Step nine: Remove and use the rest of the syrup.

If you refrigerate properly, they last 5 days.

Nutritional Information:

This is based on one pear with syrup and cinnamon

Your calories are going to be 209.7.

Your cholesterol is going to be 0 milligrams.

Your total fat is going to be 0.025 grams.

Your sodium is going to be 5.05 milligrams.

Your protein is going to be 1.05 grams.

Your total carbohydrates are going to be 53.7 grams.

Your sugar is going to be 40.65 grams.

Your fiber is going to be 6.35 grams.

Our last desert recipe is for some delicious

fruit. **Fruity Dessert**

This recipe takes only 5 minutes of prep time and 25 minutes to cook

This recipe serves 4 people

Ingredients:

- 3 tbsp of brown sugar
- 1 ½ c blueberries (make sure they are fresh)
- 1/8 tsp of cinnamon (ground)
- 4 peaches (you need to peel them and slice them)

Instructions:

- Step one: Your will need to preheat your oven to exactly 350 degrees.
- Step two: Spread the blueberries and peaches in a dish for baking.
- Step three: You need to bake this for 20 minutes.
- Step four: Turn your oven down to a low broil.
- Step five: Broil the dish for 5 minutes. (when it bubbles it is done).
- Step six: You can refrigerate and serve cold or serve warm.

Nutritional Information:

This recipe serves four, so the serving size is based on one

Your calories are going to be 90.7.

Your cholesterol is going to be 0 milligrams.

Your potassium is going to be 317.4 milligrams.

Your total fat is going to be 0.5 grams.

Your sodium is going to be 1.1 milligrams.

Your protein is going to be 1.6 grams.

Your total carbohydrates are going to be 21.95 grams.

Your sugar is going to be 19.3 grams.

Your fiber is going to be 3.2 grams.

Chapter seven: Let's Make A Meal Plan

One of the reasons that meal plans are so important is because they help you understand just what you should be eating in a day and they can help provide structure which is helpful when your trying to understand how to use this diet to achieve the best results. Remember however that it has been proven that the average adult needs at least 2,000 calories a day. These meal plans have less with the goal of losing weight in mind, but we are in no way a substitute for a professional and you should of course check with your doctor first to make sure that you can do this.

This is a seven-day meal plan that allows for two snacks as well so you shouldn't feel overly hungry as your making sure that your body gets the food it needs.

Day One:

Breakfast:

Oatmeal with pecans and berries (go for blueberries).

A medium pear.

First snack:

A cup of cucumbers (they will need to be diced).

A single tablespoon of an herb vinaigrette.

The trick to make this snack delicious is that you are going to need to toss the vegetable in the vinaigrette.

Lunch:

A medium orange.

A single serving of a veggie grain bowl with chickpeas.

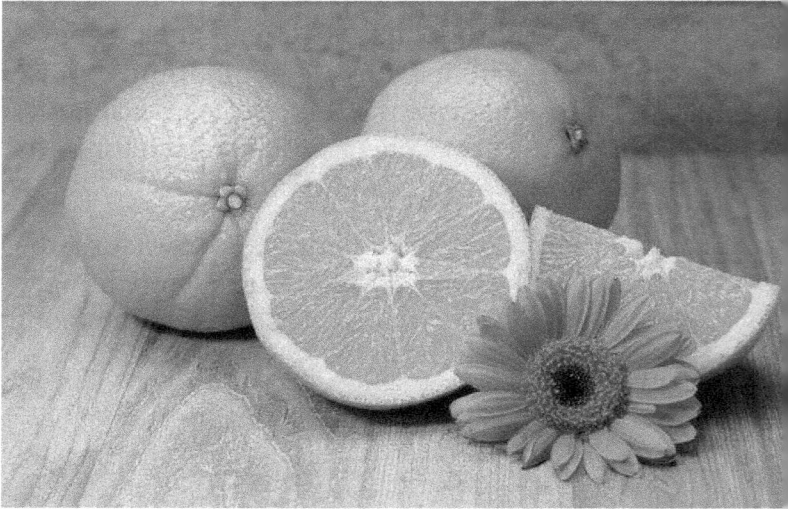

Second snack:

Carrots. You will need 2 of them and they need to be medium in size.

¼ of a cup of hummus for dipping the carrots.

Dinner:

For this one you get to eat bread. This is another thing about this diet that most appreciate.

A thick slice of a baguette (when we say thick, we don't mean a slice that's four or five inches. Try to aim for one or two inches instead).

A single serving of Orzo and Mediterranean chicken (Use a slow cooker for this).

Nutritional information for day one:

Your total calories are going to be 1,486

Your carbs are going to be 241 grams

Your fiber is going to be 41 grams

Your protein is going to be 65 grams

Your sodium is going to be 1,903

milligrams Your fat will be 36 grams

If you need to keep track of the calories at each individual meal, they are as follows.

Breakfast: 392

First snack: 60

Lunch: 364

Second snack: 154

Dinner: 516

Day Two:

Breakfast:

A single serving of raspberries with muesli

First snack:

Almonds you can have two tablespoons in this serving

Lunch:

An orange (it needs to be a medium one)

A single serving of vegetables that have been roasted and a quinoa salad

Second snack:

6-inch pita bread (you can go up to 6 ½ inches but it needs to be whole wheat)

¼ of a cup of hummus for dipping the bread

Dinner:

A single tablespoon of the vinaigrette from day one

Mixed greens to go with the vinaigrette you can have 2 cups

A single serving of gnocchi uses artichoke and tomato

Nutritional information for day two:

Your total calories are going to be 1,479

Your carbs are going to be 212 grams

Your fiber is going to be 45 grams

Your protein is going to be 50 grams

Your sodium is going to be 1,571 milligrams

Your fat will be 56 grams

If you need to keep track of the calories at each individual meal, they are as follows.

Breakfast: 287

First snack: 103

Lunch: 412

Second snack: 188

Dinner: 489

Day Three:

Breakfast:

A single serving of toast (you may use ricotta and fig)

First snack:

A serving of 2 plums

Lunch:

A medium orange.

A single serving of a salad (make sure it's green) pair this with hummus and pita bread

Second snack:

A serving of almonds (you can have 2 tablespoons)

A cup of raspberries

Dinner:

A cup of Quinoa (make sure its basic)

A single serving of salmon (make sure that its rosemary crusted with walnuts)

A cup of broccoli (make sure it's parmesan and balsamic)

Nutritional information for day three:

Your total calories are going to be 1,475

Your carbs are going to be 181 grams

Your fiber is going to be 36 grams

Your protein is going to be 71 grams

Your sodium is going to be 1,554 milligrams

Your fat will be 59 grams

If you need to keep track of the calories at each individual meal, they are as follows.

Breakfast: 252

First snack: 61

Lunch: 435

Second snack: 167

Dinner: 560

Day Four:

Breakfast:

A single serving of a frittata (go with a rainbow one today)

A medium orange

First snack:

¾ of a cup of yogurt (make sure that it's Greek and that you are using whole milk)

¾ of a cup of raspberries

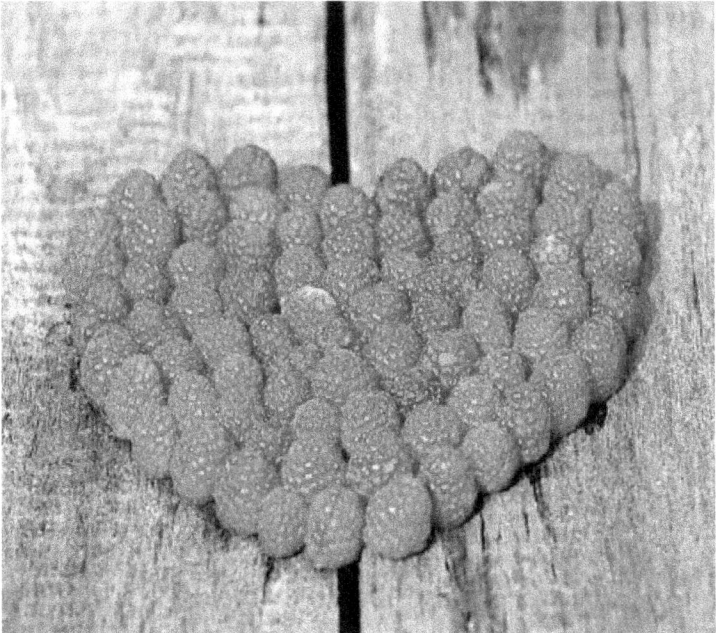

Lunch:

An herb vinaigrette (2 tablespoons)

A single serving of Orzo and Mediterranean chicken (make sure that your using a slow cooker for this)

A cup and a half of mixed greens

Second snack:

A 6 inch pita bread (you can go up another half inch but make sure it's whole wheat)

¼ of a cup of hummus for dipping the bread

Dinner:

A single serving of Salmon (Dijon) paired with a green bean pilaf

Nutritional information for day four:

Your total calories are going to be 1,525

Your carbs are going to be 123 grams

Your fiber is going to be 31 grams

Your protein is going to be 104 grams

Your sodium is going to be 1,880 milligrams

Your fat will be 71 grams

If you need to keep track of the calories at each individual meal, they are as follows.

Breakfast: 281

First snack: 233

Lunch: 381

Second snack: 188

Dinner: 442

Day Five:

Breakfast:

A single serving of toast (you may use ricotta and fig for this)

A medium orange

First snack:

A medium pear

Lunch:

A single tablespoon of the herb vinaigrette

A cup and a half of gnocchi (you may use artichoke and tomato for this)

Mixed greens (here you can have 2 cups)

Second snack:

A single tablespoon of almonds (sliced)

A cup of raspberries

A half of a cup of yogurt (make sure that it is Greek and that your using whole milk)

Dinner:

A single cup of quinoa (make sure that its basic)

A single serving of cod (serve in a cream sauce. Go for tomato cream)

Nutritional information for day one:

Your total calories are going to be 1,495

Your carbs are going to be 204 grams

Your fiber is going to be 38 grams

Your protein is going to be 68 grams

Your sodium is going to be 1,404

milligrams Your fat will be 38 grams

If you need to keep track of the calories at each individual meal, they are as follows.

Breakfast: 314

First snack: 101

Lunch: 429

Second snack: 221

Dinner: 429

Day Six:

Breakfast:

A medium orange

A single serving of muesli with berries (use Raspberries today)

First snack:

A cup of cucumbers (they will need to be

diced). A single tablespoon of an herb

vinaigrette. **Lunch:**

A thick baguette slice (when we say thick we don't mean go super thick. Go for two inches at most and one inch at least.)

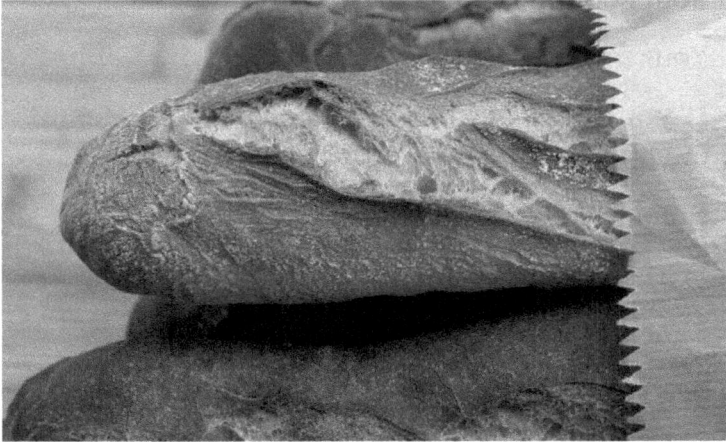

Second snack:

Hummus (you get 3 tablespoons)

6 inch pita bread (you can go up a half inch if needed but remember to use whole wheat)

Dinner:

A single serving of vegetables (roast them) with cheese (goat cheese)

Nutritional information for day six:

Your total calories are going to be 1,503

Your carbs are going to be 185 grams

Your fiber is going to be 37 grams

Your protein is going to be 87 grams

Your sodium is going to be 1,714 milligrams

Your fat will be 54 grams

If you need to keep track of the calories at each individual meal, they are as follows.

Breakfast: 349

First snack: 60

Lunch: 491

Second snack: 162

Dinner: 442

Day Seven:

For this day you will see that it's the same as day one

Breakfast:

Oatmeal with pecans and berries (go for blueberries)

A medium pear

First snack:

A cup of cucumbers (they will need to be

diced). A single tablespoon of an herb

vinaigrette. **Lunch:**

A medium orange.

A single serving of a veggie grain bowl with chickpeas.

Second snack:

Carrots. You will need 2 of them and they need to be medium in size.

¼ of a cup of hummus for dipping the carrots.

Dinner:

For this one you get to eat bread. This is another thing about this diet that most appreciate.

A thick slice of a baguette (when we say thick, we don't mean a slice that's four or five inches. Try to aim for one or two inches instead).

A single serving of Orzo and Mediterranean chicken (Use a slow cooker for this).

Nutritional information for day one:

Your total calories are going to be 1,486

Your carbs are going to be 241 grams

Your fiber is going to be 41 grams

Your protein is going to be 65 grams

Your sodium is going to be 1,903

milligrams Your fat will be 36 grams

If you need to keep track of the calories at each individual meal, they are as follows.

Breakfast: 392

First snack: 60

Lunch: 364

Second snack: 154

Dinner: 516

As you can see with this plan you get a variety of foods that are easy to make and leave you feeling satisfied but not deprived.

This next meal plan is based of a 2,000 calorie diet. Like the meal plan above we will show you the nutritional information as well. The only difference will be that we will be showing the calories so that you can see what a 2,000 calorie diet looks like.

Day one:

Breakfast: (this will be 453 in calories)

Egg toast with avocado

2 colemanites

First snack: (this will be 252 in calories)

A medium apple with peanut butter

For the peanut butter remember to only use a single tablespoon of it. If you need to go a half tablespoon higher but no more.

Lunch: (this will be 488 in calories)

Salad with greens

Hummus and pita bread

Second snack (this will be 198 in calories)

8 apricots (they need to be dried)

10 walnut halves

Dinner (this will be 589 calories)

A single cup of broccoli florets. You will need to steam them.

A single serving of chicken saltimbocca

1 ¼ of a cup of couscous. It needs to be whole wheat and cooked.

Day two:

Breakfast: (this will be 444 calories)

Oatmeal with nuts and fruit

First snack: (this will be 236 calories)

10 walnut halves

A single banana

Lunch: (this will be 477 calories)

Salad with greens paired with chickpeas that have been spiced

You can use balsamic vinegar or olive oil of course for the salad. If you do only half a tablespoon.

Second snack: (this will be 207 calories)

2 clementine's

6 inch pita bread. Be sure that its whole wheat.

2 tbsp hummus

Dinner: (this will be 639 calories)

2 cups of greens. They can be mixed for more nutrients.

2 ¼ Artichoke and Tomato Gnocchi

Day three:

Breakfast: (this will be 428 calories)

Oatmeal with nuts and fruits

1 clementine

First snack: (this will be 200 calories)

A single apple. Be sure to use a medium one.

With a single tablespoon of peanut butter

Lunch: (this will be 458 calories)

Salad with greens and chickpeas that have been spiced.

Serve with a 6 inch pita bread. Make sure its whole wheat.

Second snack: (this will be 180 calories)

2 tbsp of hummus

2 carrots. Be sure to use medium ones.

1 hardboiled egg

Dinner: (this will be 565 calories)

Salmon that has been roasted with couscous and fennel

Serve with a 6 inch pita bread. Whole wheat of course.

Third snack: (this will be 193 calories)

1 oz of chocolate. Make sure it's dark.

1 fig. Be sure its fresh and a medium size.

Day four:

Breakfast: (this will be 453 calories) Toast with banana and peanut butter **First snack: (this is 128 calories)** 2 carrots. Use medium ones. A single hardboiled egg **Lunch: (this is 488 calories)**

Salad with greens paired with hummus and pita bread

Second snack: (this is 150 calories)

1/3 of a cup of strawberries. Make sure to slice them.

1 cup of yogurt. Be sure it's plain, nonfat and Greek.

Dinner: (this is 597 calories)

A single serving of Mediterranean spinach tuna salad

Serve with 2 slices of bread. Make sure it is whole wheat and then drizzle with 1 tsp of olive oil for each slice.

Third snack: (this is 193 calories)

1 oz chocolate. Make sure it's dark.

1 single fig. Make sure that its fresh and a size medium.

Day five:

Breakfast: (this is 453 calories)

Toast with egg and avocado

2 clementine

First snack: (this is 190 calories)

7 apricots. Make sure they are dried

¼ of a cup of chickpeas that have been spiced

Lunch: (this will be 498 calories)

2 cups of greens that have been mixed

1 ½ cups of artichoke and tomato gnocchi topped with a tbsp of cheese. Use feta

Second snack: (this will 225 calories)

10 walnut halves

A single medium apple

Dinner: (this will be 626 calories)

Cod served with couscous and vegetables

Serve with pita bread. Use whole wheat and toast it.

Day six:

Breakfast: (this will be 453 calories)

Toast with banana and peanut butter

First snack: (this will be 101 calories)

A single pear. Make it a medium one.

Lunch: (this will be 480 calories)

Salad with greens paired with hummus and pita bread

Second snack: (this will be 150 calories)

1/3 of a cup of strawberries. Make sure that they are sliced.

A cup of yogurt. Make sure its Greek and plain as well as being nonfat.

Dinner: (this will be 602 calories)

2 slices of bread. Use whole wheat and drizzle with a teaspoon of olive oil

2 cups of Italian soup. This will be Egg drop.

2 cups of arugula. You will top this with a half tablespoon of olive oil

Third snack: (this will be 234 calories)

1 ½ oz of chocolate. Make sure it's dark.

Day seven:

Breakfast: (this will be 428 calories)

Oatmeal with walnuts and honey

First snack:(this will be 252 calories)

A single medium apple

1 ½ tbsp of peanut butter

Lunch: (this will be 495 calories)

2 cups of the Italian soup

1 cup of strawberries

2 cups of the arugula and olive oil

1 slice of toasted whole wheat bread

Second snack:(this will be 206 calories)

8 walnut halves

A single pear. Use a medium one.

Dinner: (this will be 637 calories)

1 ½ of a serving of Pork that has been roasted paired with a cherry tomato bowl with asparagus.

This meal plan offers more of a variety, but you can see that many of the snacks go for fruit and hummus because that is a big staple with the

Mediterranean diet and utilizing it to its full benefit.

Chapter eight: Conclusion

Many people have adopted the Mediterranean diet because they realize that there are many benefits that they can utilize from adopting this healthy lifestyle. The recipes in this book make it even easier because we've given you a handful of recipes for every meal and gone even further by offering two differing meal plans and desserts as well as snacks. We've also taught you that you can still eat your favorite foods instead of giving them up completely. The only thing you have to do is be smarter about how you make your food and the recipes that you use to your advantage. No matter the calorie intake that you've set for yourself with this diet you can eat great tasting food that not only makes you feel well but is healthy for you.

Many people find that when they are starting a diet they don't know which recipes they need to use and what they need to buy. Through this book, you haven been able to utilize healthy recipes and learn new flavor combinations from amazing cultures that are renowned for their food. The meal plan also has many ideas of food that you should be thinking about eating and how to prepare them. if your someone who doesn't like to cook your in luck here as well because we have included many different recipes that serve at least 6 people. If you live alone or don't have children, voilà! Left overs and meals that you can take on the go and use for your benefit. This diet also offers ingredients that in other diet's you would have to avoid but, in this diet,, you can utilize for the benefits they offer. The same is true for some of the food you will find you need to eat on this diet as well.

Examples of what we mean are olive oil for one because it can be high in fat. Other diets won't let you eat this for that very reason and try and have you avoided it entirely. This diet has you eating a lot of olive oil (although you should remember the moderation rule because that is important for any diet that you undertake). Another example is that other diet's say that you can't have fish because they believe it's harmful. This diet is the opposite and encourages you to eat a lot of fish because it realizes that fish is healthy for you because of all the vitamins and minerals that they contain. In fact, for the Mediterranean diet, you are encouraged to eat mostly fish and less meat of other kinds.

Utilizing eating habits from different countries and learning how to make new dishes is going to be a great way for you to get healthy and understand what it is you have to do for your body and for yourself. By learning more things about how other cultures you get a broader sense of health and the benefits that you can receive. Many other cultures have a longer lifespan and they have been able to stay energized and healthy and we can take a page out of their book and learn from them.

Wean see what they are doing right and in turn what we are doing wrong. You can also learn how to shop better because this diet requires more fresh food and asks that you're staying away from processed foods. This is turn will help your finances and help you be able to buy the healthy food that you need on this diet. This diet is not only good for your body but it's also good for your heart and your mind. This means that you can reap the benefits of this diet safely and securely and make sure that you're lowering your risk of an early death which is the greatest achievement of any diet.

Description

Many diets have been around the block and couldn't stand the test of time. The Mediterranean diet breaks them all because it's here to stay and has been for years. It offers healthy benefits and almost no negative side effects have been shown from using this diet. However, this book shows both the pros and very few cons of this diet to give you a conclusive overview so that you can make the best decision for yourself as well as being able to be more informed. Obviously, you would need to check with your doctor to be sure that this diet is for you because this book is in no way a substitute for a medical professional.

However, studies have shown that the Mediterranean diet has been shown to be able to help your heart and your mind as well. Because of the nature of the food that you will be eating this diet also boasts that it can help prevent neurodegenerative diseases as well. In recent years research has been ongoing about whether or not this diet could have an impact in helping depression. This diet is amazing because of its ability to try and heal your mind along with your body.

With incredible food and influence from Greece, Italy, and Spain, the Mediterranean diet has a rich culture of food and it has thousands of recipes that you can peruse at your disposal. Many people don't even know where to begin and that's where this book comes in. In this book, we've taken a lot of the guesswork out for you and included breakfast recipes, lunch recipes, dinner recipes, snack recipes, and even dessert recipes. Each recipe opens you up to the culture and different styles of eating as well as using a variety of ingredients. We've thought outside of the box and listed recipes that you can enjoy anytime and anywhere as well as making sure that they are family friendly. You may be surprised to find family favorites such as turkey burgers and pizza in the mix because in this diet you don't have to give them up. You just need to make sure that your eating smarter. For fans of pudding and sweet treats, you may be surprised to see them in this book as well. No matter what your craving we have got you covered with over 30 recipes to explore.

To show you just what the Mediterranean diet looks like we've even gone further and included two separate meal plans for you in this book. Both are for seven days and show you three meals and two snacks. It also calculates the caloric intake for you and shows the nutritional information broken down step by step so that it is super simple to understand and won't leave you confused. With all of this information at your feet, you can't go wrong. This is the perfect book for beginners to understand the Mediterranean diet and begin to learn how to make amazing recipes for themselves.